28-DAYS WORKOUT CHALLENGE FOR SENIORS

Build confidence and strength with this tailored challenge featuring balance exercises, upper body strength building, lower body sculpting, and core engagement workouts.

RICHARD E. MARSHALL

GET ACCESS TO MY MORE FITNESS BOOKS

CONTENTS:

INTRODUCTIONS

Have you ever glanced in the mirror and seen a vivid, dynamic spirit aching to break free? To rediscover the joy of exercise, the excitement of exceeding your limitations, and the assurance that comes with knowing you're in control of your own health? If so, join us on this 28-day adventure where age is only a number and constraints are nothing but stepping stones.

This isn't just a workout; it's a revolution. An opportunity to alter the story that says "age equals decline." We're here to say, with every step, stretch, and drop of sweat, that life beyond 50 is a blank canvas ripe for the brilliant colors of health, happiness, and new possibilities. Forget gym subscriptions and rigorous workout regimes. This is your personal fitness studio, made in the privacy of your own home, using your own body as the instrument. We'll harness the power of basic, effective workouts that target every muscle, bone, and joint without jarring impact or overcomplicating things. Chairs morph into strong companions, walls become push-up havens, and your own body weight becomes your most powerful instrument.

Consider waking up with a spring in your step rather than a grumble in your back. Consider ascending stairs without stumbling and laughing with grandkids without gasping for air. Consider the confidence that exudes from within you as you move through your everyday duties with greater ease and elegance. This is the promise of this 28-day challenge, my buddy.

However, it is not only about the physical. This trip is a holistic symphony in which every note corresponds to your whole well-being. We'll incorporate gentle stretches to relieve tension, mindfulness techniques to quiet the mind, and even lighthearted games that promote laughter and social connection.

Forget about the dread of falling and the concern about "being too old." We'll walk with purpose, respect for our bodies, and the steadfast conviction that every stride forward is a success. We'll create a supportive community by encouraging one another, sharing tips and achievements, and demonstrating that age is only a number when we're joined by a common enthusiasm for ourselves and our well-being.

This is not a quick repair; it is a change. We'll arm you with the knowledge and confidence to continue making good choices after the following 28 days. We'll inspire you to dance with your own body for the rest of your life. So, are you prepared? Are you ready to free yourself from the constraints of preconceived conceptions and take your proper place as a dynamic, active part of life's magnificent orchestra?

Then go on this 28-day journey in which aging fades into the background and the melody of your revitalized energy takes center stage. Let us move together, laugh together, and show ourselves and the world that life beyond 50 is a beautiful ascension rather than an elegant decline.

Open the book, open your heart, and prepare to be surprised by a world of possibilities. It's your age. This is your chance. This is your 28-day road to becoming ageless.

Why every senior needs this 28-day dose of exercise

As a fitness trainer for over a decade, I've seen many transformations, but none more amazing than those in our older groups. Why? Because fitness is more than just chiselled biceps and ripped abs to them. It's about recovering one's freedom, embracing life's opportunities, and rewriting one's own aging story. Before you respond, "Oh, I couldn't possibly..." consider this. It's not about climbing mountains or breaking Olympic records. It's about taking 28 days to rediscover your own body's potential, and here's why it is important:

1. Balance:

Consider traversing your house with confidence rather than terror. Regular exercise enhances proprioception, the internal GPS that keeps you upright and helps you avoid falls, which are the greatest cause of injury in seniors. Stronger leg muscles, stronger core engagement, and superior reflexes all contribute to that smooth, firm stride, helping you to handle stairs, uneven terrain, and life's unexpected bumps with renewed confidence.

2. Strength:

Remember how easy it was to climb trees when you were a kid? That strength isn't gone; it's simply dormant. Exercise wakes it up, allowing you to create lean muscular mass that allows you to carry groceries, open heavy doors, and even tend to your garden. Consider lifting your grandkids with a giggle rather than a sigh, or accomplishing housework without breaking a sweat. Strength isn't only about vanity; it's about daily independence and the satisfaction of knowing you're competent.

3. Adaptability:

Remember how you could bend without suffering to tie your shoes? Gentle stretches and yoga positions, in particular, keep your joints lubricated and your muscles flexible. Increased mobility entails reaching for high shelves without using a ladder, tying your laces with a grin, and enjoying a pain-free morning stretch that gives you a boost of energy to start the day. It's a minor miracle in and of itself, rewriting the script of age-related stiffness and opening the door to a life of unrestricted movement.

4. Mood:

Forget about taking drugs to obtain that extra pep in your stride. Exercise is a natural mood enhancer since it increases endorphins, the brain's own feel-good chemicals. It relieves tension and anxiety while leaving you feeling invigorated and cheerful. Imagine waking up with a spring in your step, finding delight in ordinary tasks, and approaching obstacles with newfound vigor. Exercise isn't only about improving your physical health; it's also about improving your mental health and painting your life with brilliant hues of optimism.

But wait, isn't exercise hazardous to the health of seniors?

Certainly not! In fact, a personalized workout regimen, such as the one we'll be embarking on, is precisely developed to be safe and beneficial for people of various fitness levels. We'll start with mild warm-ups, then move on to low-impact exercises, gradually increasing intensity while keeping your comfort and restrictions in mind. Forget about high-pressure workouts and dangerous gym equipment. This is about moving with delight, honoring your physique's rhythm, and appreciating every tiny triumph along the road.

One day at a time, embrace this transformation.

These 28 days will be about more than simply burning calories; they will be about starting a new chapter in your life. You'll discover a strength you didn't know you possessed, a tenacity that takes you by surprise, and a renewed delight in movement. You'll be astounded at how fast your body responds, your self-confidence rises, and your spirit dances to the beat of your own revitalized vigor.

So, are you up for this trip with me? Remember that age is just a number, and your body is an amazing machine just waiting to be found. Let's spend the next 28 days rewriting the screenplay, moving with purpose, and painting the canvas of your life with brilliant hues of strength, flexibility, and joy. It's time to reclaim your freedom, embrace the possibilities, and demonstrate that life, after all, begins when you make the choice to start moving!

Are you ready to dive in? Let's get ready for the following chapter, in which you will become the creator of your own fitness romance.

CHAPTER 1

Week 1: Balance and Coordination Workouts

Welcome to the first week of your 28-Day Challenge! This week, we'll concentrate on Balance and Coordination, which will provide the groundwork for better stability and confidence in your movements. Always listen to your body, alter workouts as required, and have fun!

Weeks	Focus Area	Warm-Up (5minute)	Daily Focus Workout (25minute)	Cool-Down (5 minutes)
1: Balance & Coordination	Improve stability and control	Gentle arm circles, leg swings, neck rolls	Tai Chi exercises, standing balance poses, walking with variations (backward, side steps)	Gentle stretches for legs, back, and neck

2: Upper Body Strength	Build strength in arms, chest, and back	Arm circles, leg swings, gentle shoulder rolls	Chair dips, reverse flyes, arm circles with overhead reach, wall sit with bicep curls, can opener exercise	Stretches for biceps, triceps, shoulders, and chest
3: Lower Body Strength & Flexibility	Strengthen legs and improve flexibility	Leg swings, foot circles, arm circles	Squats, lunges, heel raises, side leg lifts (standing or lying down), step-ups (chair or stairs)	Hamstring, quad, calf, and piriformis stretches
4: Core Engagement & Cardio	Strengthen core and boost heart health	Gentle arm circles, marching in place, neck rolls	Marching with knee lifts, plank variations, walking lunges with torso twist, wall	Chest, hamstring, quad, and arm stretches

			sit with leg lifts, chair dance party	

5-minute warm-up:

Gentle arm circles: 10 forward circles, 10 backward circles for each arm.

Leg swings: 10 swings forward and 10 swings back for each leg.

5 slow rolls clockwise, 5 slow rolls anti-clockwise on the neck.

Workout (25 minutes):

Single-leg stance balance

Steps:

1. Place your feet hip-width apart and stand tall. For balance, extend your arms out to the sides.
2. Slowly raise one leg off the ground and hold for 5 seconds. Maintain a strong core and a sturdy standing leg.

3. Rep on the opposite side. Aim for three sets of five reps per leg.

Modification: If standing on one leg is too difficult, hang onto a chair or a wall for support.

Walking in tandem coordination

Steps:

1. Place your feet hip-width apart and stand tall.
2. Put one foot in front of the other, heel to toe.
3. Maintain your equilibrium by taking short, deliberate steps forward. Walk for 10 meters or as far as you can tolerate.
4. Return in the other way by turning around. Strive to complete two sets.

Modification: Shorten your steps or lean on a wall for support if necessary.

Heel-toe walk balance

Steps:

1. Stand tall, feet hip-width apart.
2. Lift one foot's heel off the ground and touch your toes to the floor behind you.

3. Return your heel to the starting position slowly and repeat with the opposite foot.
4. For 10 meters or as tolerated, walk forward or backward in this heel-toe rhythm. Attempt to complete two sets.

Modification: You can perform the exercise in situ or with support from a chair or wall.

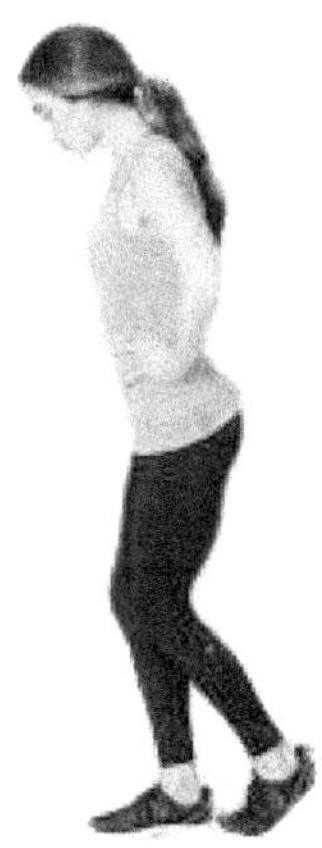

Chair Tai Chi (balance and coordination when sitting)

Steps:

1. Sit up straight on a chair, feet flat on the floor, back straight.
2. Spread your arms out to the sides, palms down.

3. As if you were carrying a ball in each hand, softly roll your arms forward, circling them at shoulder height. Rep in the other direction.
4. Gently rotate your torso from side to side, each time glancing over your shoulder.
5. Raise one leg slowly off the ground, hold for 3 seconds, then drop it back down. Rep with the opposite leg.
6. Aim for 10 repetitions of each movement in two sets of ten.

Modification: Use a lower chair or lean your back against a wall if sitting upright is uncomfortable for you.

Flamingo Stand Challenge

Steps:

1. Stand tall with your feet hip-width apart.
2. Balance on one leg while lifting the other off the ground.
3. For balance, stretch your arms out to the sides. Hold for 5-10 seconds before switching legs.
4. Strive for three sets of five reps per leg.

Modification: You can grab onto a chair or wall for support if standing on one leg is too difficult for you. Do the exercise with both feet level on the ground, elevating one leg slightly behind you for a few seconds at a time.

Stork Walk Coordination

Steps:

1. Take a tall stance with your feet hip-width apart.
2. Balance on one leg and extend the other straight out in front of you.
3. Keep your extended leg parallel to the floor and your toes pointed.
4. Maintain your equilibrium by taking short, deliberate steps forward. Walk for 10 meters or as far as you can tolerate.
5. Rep with the opposite leg. Attempt to complete two sets.

Modification: Shorten your steps or grab a chair or a wall for support if necessary. You may also perform the exercise while standing, elevating one leg and holding it for a few seconds at a time.

Side Stepping Balance

Steps:

1. Stand with your feet hip-width apart and tall.
2. To the side, take short steps, first with one foot and then bringing the other foot beside it.
3. Maintain your body's uprightness and core engagement.

4. Walk in either direction sideways for ten meters, or as permitted. Attempt to complete two sets.

Modification: Hold on to a chair or a wall for support if necessary. You may also lessen your steps or do the workout at a slower pace.

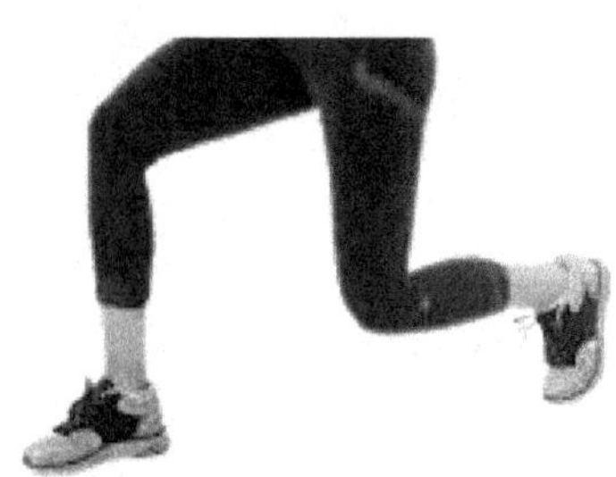

Balance of Clock Rotation

Steps:

1. For balance, stand tall with your feet hip-width apart and your arms out to the sides.
2. Consider the floor to be a clock face.
3. Slowly "walk" around the clock face, beginning at 12 o'clock and working clockwise.
4. As you take each stride, maintain your torso erect and your feet rotating together.
5. Make one full circle, then the other direction. Attempt to complete two sets.

Modification: If necessary, reduce the steps or make the clock face smaller. You can also use a chair or a wall for support.

Ball Toss Coordination

Steps:

1. Hold a tiny, soft ball in your hands and stand tall with your feet hip-width apart.
2. Throw the ball into the air and grab it with both hands.
3. Repeat, but this time try to catch the ball with only one hand.
4. You may also toss the ball to yourself and catch it with the other hand.
5. Each variant should be repeated 10 times.

Modification: Use a bigger ball or begin by bouncing the ball on the floor rather than tossing it up.

Ladder Drill Footwork

Steps:

1. Locate a ladder on a level area or draw two lines of tape on the floor to make your own ladder.
2. Step one foot into the first square of the ladder.
3. Step into the next square with your other foot behind you.
4. Step forward and backward through the ladder, concentrating on strong footwork and synchronization.
5. Repeat the ladder 5 times in either direction. Attempt to complete two sets.

Modification: Make the ladder squares bigger or climb through the ladder sideways if necessary.

Sensory Foot Exploration

Steps:

1. Take your shoes and socks off.
2. Stand on various surfaces, such as a soft rug, a lumpy mat, or even outside on the grass.
3. Pay attention to how your feet feel on each surface and adjust your balance as needed.
4. Slowly walk across each surface, paying attention to the various sensations.
5. Give each surface 5 minutes.

Modification: If necessary, you can perform this exercise while wearing shoes.

Seated Leg Twists Rotation

Steps:

1. Sit up straight on a chair, feet flat on the floor, back straight.
2. Position your hands on your knees.
3. Twist your torso slowly from side to side, each time glancing over your shoulder.
4. Maintain a strong core and a straight back.
5. Do two sets of 10 repetitions on each side.

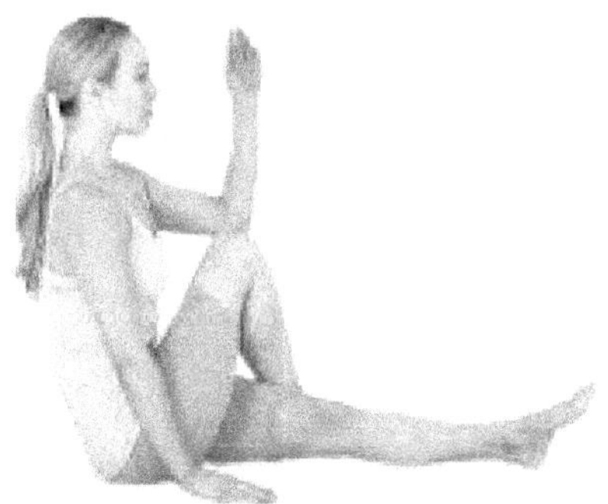

5 minutes Cool-down

- Stretching gently: Hold each stretch for 30 seconds.
- Stretch your hamstrings by sitting on the floor with one leg extended and the other bowed. Lean forward toward your outstretched leg.
- Stand tall and balance by holding onto a chair or a wall. Bend one leg behind you and gently bring your heel towards your buttocks by grabbing your foot (or using a strap if necessary).
- Calf stretch: Face a wall with your hands shoulder-width apart on the wall. Lean forward, keeping your heels level on the ground, until your calves stretch.

CHAPTER 2

Week 2: Upper Body Strength Workouts

Hello and welcome to Week 2 of your 28-Day Challenge! This week, we'll focus on your upper body strength, muscular growth, and overall capacity to manage daily chores with ease. Always listen to your body, alter workouts as required, and have fun!

5-minute warm-up:

Gentle arm circles: 10 forward circles, 10 backward circles for each arm.

neck roll: 5 slow rolls clockwise, 5 slow rolls anticlockwise

Shoulder shrugs are performed by rolling your shoulders up towards your ears, holding for a second, and then relaxing. Rep 10 times more.

Workout (25 minutes)

Wall push-ups

Steps:

1. Stand with your feet shoulder-width apart, facing a wall.
2. Place your hands shoulder-width apart at chest height on the wall.
3. Bend your elbows and drop your chest slowly towards the wall, maintaining your back straight and your core engaged.
4. Push up to return to the starting position.
5. Strive for three sets of eight to twelve repetitions per set.

Modification: Start with your hands higher on the wall, or execute the exercise from your knees.

Bicep curls (light weights or water bottles)

Steps:

1. Hold a weight or a water bottle in each hand while you stand tall with your feet hip-width apart.
2. Bend your elbows and bring the weights up to your shoulders.
3. Slowly return the weights to their initial position.
4. Strive for three sets of 10-15 reps.

Modification: Use less weight or do the workout without weights.

Tricep extensions (light weights or water bottles)

Steps:

1. Hold a weight or a water bottle in each hand above and stand tall with your feet hip-width apart.
2. Bend your elbows while keeping your elbows close to your head and lowering the weights behind your head.
3. Slowly return your arms to that initial position.
4. Make three sets of 10-15 repetitions each.
5. Use less weight or do the workout without weights.

Modification: Use less weight or do the exercise without weights.

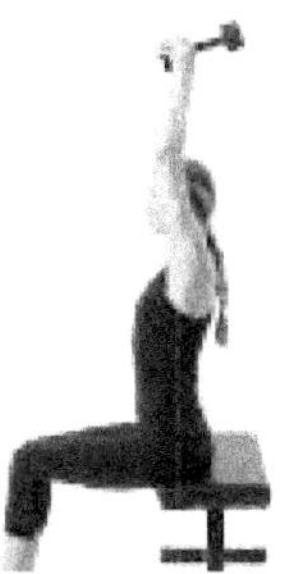

Seated Rows (resistance band or towel)

Steps:

1. Sit up straight on a chair, feet flat on the floor, back straight.

2. Wrap a resistance band or cloth behind you around a doorknob or other secure item.
3. Squeeze your shoulder blades together as you bring your elbows down towards your sides, holding the band or towel in each hand.
4. Return your arms to the starting position slowly.
5. Perform three sets of 10-15 repetitions each.

Modification: Use a lighter resistance band or do the exercise without resistance.

Overhead press (light weights or water bottles)

Steps:

1. Stand tall with your feet hip-width apart and a weight or water bottle in each hand at shoulder height.
2. Maintaining core engagement, raise your arms straight up overhead.
3. Return the weights to shoulder height gradually.
4. Aim for three sets of eight to twelve repetitions.

Modification: Use less weight or do the workout without weights.

Chair Dipping

Steps:

1. Place your feet level on the floor and your hands shoulder-width apart on the seat's edge.
2. Slide forward till your hands are almost off the edge of the chair and your fingers grab the front of it.
3. Slowly bend your elbows and lower your body until your knees create a 90-degree angle.
4. Return to the starting position by pushing up.
5. Aim for three sets of eight to twelve repetitions.

Modification: If chair dips are too difficult, try modified dips with your hands on a higher surface, such as a table or countertop.

Reverse Flyes (seated or standing)

Steps:

1. Place your feet hip-width apart, sit up straight, and hold a water bottle or small weight in each hand while extending your arms to shoulder height.
2. Spread your arms to the sides slowly, maintaining your back straight and your core engaged.
3. At the top of the exercise, squeeze your shoulder blades together.
4. Return your arms to their original positions.

5. Strive for three sets of 10-15 repetitions per set.

Modification: Use lesser weights or do the workout without weights. You may even perform it while sitting for increased support.

Overhead Reach Arm Circles

Steps:

1. Maintain a tall stance, place your feet hip-width apart, and raise your arms to shoulder height, palms down.
2. Make little circles with your arms, gradually increasing their size.
3. Reach your arms aloft, palms facing each other, after a few rotations. Hold for a few of seconds.
4. Return your arms to the beginning position and complete the circles in the other way.
5. Strive for three sets of ten circles in each direction.

Modification: If necessary, make smaller circles or forgo the overhead reach.

Wall Sit with Bicep Curls

Steps:

1. Face a wall and lean back until your back is flat against it and your knees are bent at a 90-degree angle, as if sitting in a chair.
2. Hold light weights or water bottles at your sides in each hand.
3. Curl your arms up towards your shoulders, then lower them slowly back down.
4. Maintain the wall sit position while performing bicep curls.
5. Hold the wall sit comfortably for at least 30 seconds.

Modification: If holding the wall sit for 30 seconds is too difficult, try with shorter holds and progressively increase the length as your strength improves. You may also practice the bicep curls without weights or while sitting on a chair rather than against a wall.

Can Opener Exercise (light weights or water bottles)

Steps:

1. Stand tall, feet hip-width apart, and hold small weights or water bottles in each hand, arms stretched overhead, palms front.
2. Descend your arms slowly down and across your body, as if opening a can with a can opener, until your elbows almost meet at your sides.

3. Reverse the movement by raising your arms
   overhead again.
4. Strive for three sets of 10-15 repetitions per set.

Modification: Use lesser weights or do the workout
without weights. You might alternatively begin with your
arms slightly bent at the elbows rather than fully stretched
above.

Bonus: Add resistance bands to any of these workouts for
an added challenge!

5 minutes Cool-down

- Stretching gently: Hold each stretch for 30 seconds.
- Raise your arm upward with your elbow bent and
  grip your elbow with your other hand to stretch your
  triceps. Pull your elbow behind your head gently.
- Stretch your chest by clasping your hands behind
  your back and gently pulling your shoulders back.
- Tilt your head to one side and gently rest your ear on
  your shoulder to lengthen your neck. Hold for 30
  seconds before switching sides.

CHAPTER 3

Week 3: Lower Body Strength and Flexibility Workouts

Hello and welcome to Week 3 of your 28-Day Challenge! This week, we'll focus on your lower body, strengthening and stretching your legs and core. Always listen to your body, alter workouts as required, and have fun!

5-minute warm-up:

- Gentle leg swings: 10 swings forward and ten swings back for each leg.
- Foot circles: Make 10 clockwise and 10 counter clockwise circles with your feet for each ankle.
- Arm circles: 10 forward circles, 10 backward circles for each arm.

25 minutes Workout

Squats

Steps:

1. With your toes pointing slightly outward and your feet hip-width apart, take a tall stance.
2. Maintain a straight back and engaged core as you bend your knees as if sitting in a chair.
3. Bend yourself until your thighs are parallel to the floor (or as low as you feel comfortable), then push yourself back up to the starting position.
4. Strive for three sets of eight to twelve repetitions.

Modification: Hold onto a chair or a wall for support, or perform chair squats by sitting and standing on a solid chair.

Lunges

Steps:

1. Place your feet hip-width apart and stand tall.
2. Step forward on one leg, lowering your hips until your knees are at 90-degree angles.
3. Return to the beginning position and do the same with the other leg.
4. Go for three sets of eight to twelve repetitions each leg.

Modification: Take fewer steps or reduce the depth of your lunges, or conduct stationary lunges by putting one foot forward without lowering your hips.

Heel raises

Steps:

1. Standing tall with your feet hip-width apart, raise your heels off the ground and balance on the balls of your feet.
2. Hold for a few seconds before dropping your heels softly.
3. Strive for three sets of 15-20 reps.

Modification: Hold on to a chair or a wall for support, or do calf lifts while standing on a step or curb.

Hamstring stretch (sitting)

Steps:

1. Place your legs out in front of you while sitting on the floor.
2. Bend forward from your hips, stretching your hands as far as you can to your toes.
3. Maintain the stretch for 30 seconds.
4. Rep on the opposite side.

Modification: Use a strap or cloth to assist you reach your toes, or sit with your legs bent if necessary.

Quad stretch (standing)

Steps:

1. To keep your equilibrium, stand up and grab a chair or a wall.
2. Bend one leg behind you and gently bring your heel towards your buttocks by grabbing your foot (or using a strap if necessary).
3. Maintain the stretch for 30 seconds.
4. Rep on the opposite side.

Modification: Do the stretch without holding your foot against the wall, or avoid the exercise if it causes pain.

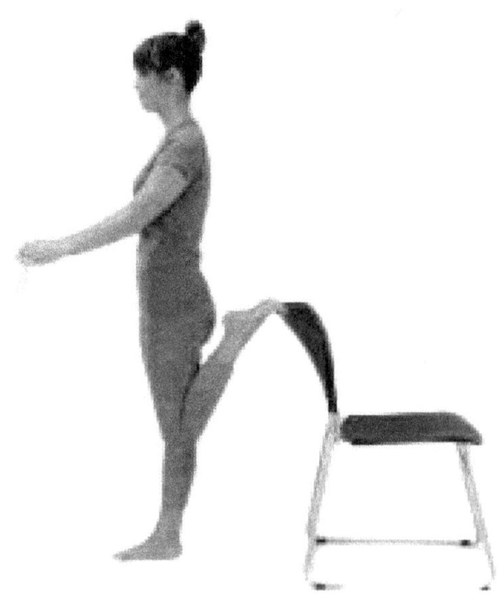

Side leg lifts (standing or lying down)

Steps:

1. As you stand, place your feet hip-width apart and, if necessary, grab on to a chair or the wall for support. Lift one leg out to the side slowly, keeping your hips square and your core engaged. Before lowering it, hold it for a few seconds. Rep on the opposite side.
2. When you're lying down, stack your legs on your side. Lift your upper leg toward the ceiling while maintaining your hips steady. Before lowering it, hold it for a few seconds. Rep on the opposite side.

Modification: Do lesser leg lifts or lessen the hold period, or merely touch your foot off the ground instead of fully raising it.

Step-ups (from a chair or the stairs)

Steps:

1. Locate a solid chair or step that is around knee-height.
2. Step one leg onto the chair, then bring the second leg up to join it.
3. Return to the beginning position and do the same with the other leg.

4. Strive for three sets of eight to twelve repetitions each leg.

Modification: Use a lower chair or step for support, or hang onto a railing. You may also perform the exercise without standing up by elevating one leg at a time.

Wall sits

Steps:

1. Face a wall and lean back until your back is flat against it and your knees are bent at a 90-degree angle, as if sitting in a chair.
2. Maintain the position for as long as you can comfortably do so, aiming for at least 30 seconds.

Modification: If holding the wall sit for 30 seconds is too difficult, start with shorter holds and progressively increase the length as you gain strength. You may also use a chair instead of the wall.

Figure-four stretch

Steps:

1. Rest on your back, legs bent, feet flat on the floor.

2. Cross one ankle slightly above the knee over the opposing thigh.
3. Pull the crossed knee to your chest gently until you feel a stretch in your glutes and piriformis.
4. Maintain the stretch for 30 seconds.
5. Rep on the opposite side.

Modification: Use a strap or towel to assist draw your knee closer together, or omit the exercise if it causes pain.

Calf raises with variations

Steps:

1. Calf rises on one leg: Take a tall stance on one leg and elevate your heel off the floor. Hold it for a few seconds before lowering it. Rep with the other leg.
2. Ball wall calf raises: Stand with your hands shoulder-width apart, facing a wall, and insert a tiny ball between your calves. Lean forward, forcing your heels into the ball until your calves stretch. Before releasing, hold for a few seconds.

Modification: Calf rises with both fcct flat on the ground can be modified, or you can grasp onto a chair or a wall for support.

Add weights to your lunges or step-ups for an added challenge, or try leg lifts and side steps with resistance bands around your ankles.

Cool-down (5 minutes):

- Stretching gently: Hold each stretch for 30 seconds.
- Calf stretch: Face a wall with your hands shoulder-width apart on the wall. Lean forward, keeping your heels level on the ground, until your calves stretch.
- Sit on the floor with your feet together and your knees bent outward for an inner thigh stretch. Gently push your knees on the floor.
- Stretch your piriformis by lying on your back with your knees bent and your feet flat on the floor. Cross one ankle slightly above the knee over the opposing thigh. Pull the crossed knee to your chest gently until you feel a stretch in your buttocks.

Remember that this is only a sample workout. Feel free to combine workouts, change the intensity, and take rest days as required. The most essential thing is to get your body moving, have fun, and celebrate your accomplishments!

Wear comfortable shoes and clothes that allows you to move freely.

CHAPTER 4

Week 4: Core Engagement and Cardio Workouts

Welcome to Week 4 of your 28-Day Challenge! This week, we'll focus on core engagement and cardio to improve your heart health, stability, and general endurance. Remember to listen to your body, alter workouts as required, and, most importantly, enjoy yourself!

5-minute warm-up:

- Gentle arm circles: 10 forward circles, 10 backward circles for each arm.
- Leg swings: ten swings forward and ten swings back for each leg.
- 5 slow rolls clockwise, 5 slow rolls counterclockwise on the neck.

Workout (25 minutes):

Marching with knee lifts

Steps:

1. Maintain a tall posture with your feet hip-width apart and your core engaged.
2. March in place, raising your knees as high as you can comfortably.
3. March with your arms naturally swinging.
4. Maintain proper posture and controlled movements for 2 minutes.

Modification: March in place without elevating your knees, or lower the height of your knee lifts.

Plank variations

Steps:

1. Begin in a high plank posture, with your hands shoulder width apart and your body straight from head to heels.
2. Maintain for 30 seconds, being sure to engage your core and maintain your hips level.
3. Try a kneeling plank on your knees or a forearms plank with your elbows bent and squarely under your shoulders for a modified version.
4. Repeat the plank hold three times, taking small breaks in between.

Modification: Start with shorter plank holds or lower yourself to your knees or elbows.

Walking lunges with torso twist

Steps:

1. Stand with your feet hip-width apart and tall.
2. Move forward with one leg, dropping your hips and bringing your other knee to the floor.
3. Twist your torso slightly towards the front leg as you lunge.
4. Return to the initial position and repeat on the other side.
5. Set a goal of 10 repetitions each leg.

Modification: Change it up by doing lesser lunges or skipping the torso twist.

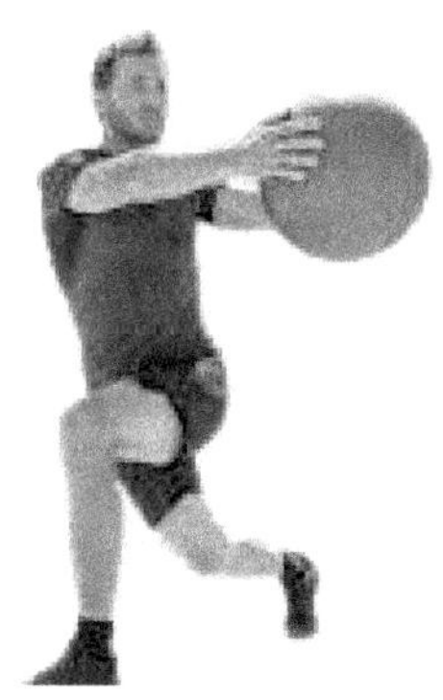

Wall sit with leg raises

Steps:

1. Face a wall and lean back until your back is flat against it and your knees are bent at a 90-degree angle, as if sitting in a chair.
2. Lift one leg off the ground while maintaining your core tight and your hips square.
3. Before lowering it, hold it for a few seconds.
4. Rep on the opposite side.
5. Aim for 10 reps each leg, each held for 3 seconds.

Modification: Hold on to a chair or a wall for support, or skip the leg lifts and simply sit on the wall.

Chair dance party

Steps:

1. Place your feet flat on the floor and sit on a solid chair.
2. Put on some upbeat music and have fun! Dance in your chair by moving your arms, twisting your torso, tapping your feet, and tapping your feet.
3. Have fun and be creative! Continue for another 5 minutes.
4. Sit with your back to the chair for more support, or simply tap your feet and sway to the music.

March with arm circles

Steps:

1. Maintain a tall posture with your feet hip-width apart and your core engaged.
2. March in place, raising your knees as high as you can comfortably.
3. Swing your arms in huge circles, one forward and one backward, at the same time.
4. Maintain proper posture and controlled movements for 2 minutes.

Modification: Reduce the size of your arm circles or march in place without elevating your knees.

Bird-dog

Steps:

1. Start on all fours with your hands shoulder-width apart and your knees hip-width apart.
2. Keep your back straight and your core taut.
3. Maintain a neutral spine by extending one arm forward and the opposing leg back at the same moment.
4. Hold for a few seconds, then return to your starting position and do the opposite side.
5. Aim for ten reps on each side.

Modification: Start on your knees or forearms, or reduce the length of your arm and leg reach.

Side-stepping with torso twist

Steps:

1. With your feet hip-width apart and your arms out to the sides at shoulder height, take a proud stance.
2. Take a modest right-side stride, rotating your torso slightly in the direction you're going.
3. Bring your left foot alongside your right, then switch sides, turning your body to the left.
4. Continue to sidestep and twist for 1 minute.

Modification: Reduce the amount of your steps or omit the torso twist.

Chair leg extensions with twist

Steps:

1. Place your feet flat on the floor and your hands on your thighs while sitting in a firm chair.
2. Maintain your core engaged and your spine straight by extending one leg straight out in front of you.
3. Twist your body slightly to the same side as you extend your leg.

4. Hold for a few seconds, then return to your starting position and do the opposite side.
5. Set a goal of 10 repetitions each leg.

Modification: skip the torso twist and perform the exercise with shorter leg extensions.

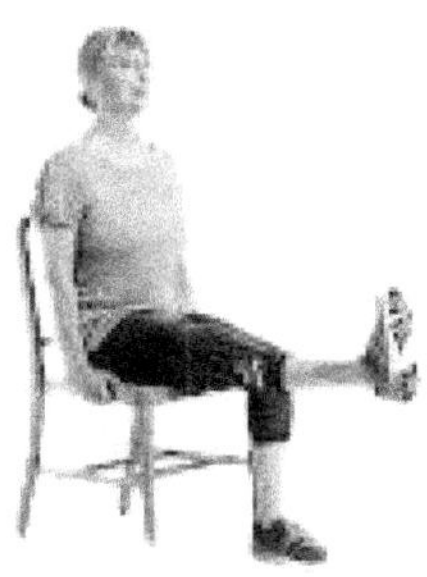

Quick feet with the chair

Steps:

1. Place your feet flat on the floor and your hands on your thighs while sitting in a firm chair.
2. Lift your heels off the ground slightly and tap your toes up and down for 30 seconds.
3. Maintain core engagement and prevent bouncing in your chair.

Modification: Tap your toes more slowly or omit the heel lift.

Bonus: You may add weights to your leg lifts when doing wall sits or knee lifts while marching for an added challenge. Interval training, in which you alternate high-intensity activities like jumping jacks or stair climbing with times of recovery walking, is another option.

5 minutes Cool-down

- Stretching gently: Hold each stretch for 30 seconds.
- Stretch your hamstrings by sitting on the floor with one leg extended and the other bowed. Lean forward toward your outstretched leg.
- Stand tall and balance by holding onto a chair or a wall. Bend one leg behind you and gently bring your heel towards your buttocks by grabbing your foot (or using a strap if necessary).
- Stretch your chest by clasping your hands behind your back and gently pulling your shoulders back.

Consider include moderate-intensity cardio exercises such as swimming, bicycling, or walking outside in your weekly regimen to get extra heart health advantages.

CHAPTER 5

Dietary Recommendations

Focus on balanced meals: Each meal should contain carbs, protein, and healthy fats to give long-lasting energy and to aid in muscle development and repair.

Make whole foods a priority: Over processed foods, choose fresh fruits and vegetables, whole grains, lean protein sources, and healthy fats like nuts and seeds.

Hydrate properly: To keep hydrated and maintain healthy bodily function, drink enough of water throughout the day. Every day, drink 8-10 glasses of water.

Reduce your intake of added sweets and harmful fats: To maintain a healthy heart and body weight, avoid sugary beverages, fried meals, and processed meats.

Pay attention to your body: Eat when you're hungry and quit when you're satisfied. Pay heed to your body's cues and make appropriate eating choices.

Consult a medical professional: Before beginning any new exercise or nutritional program, consult with your doctor or registered dietitian about your individual health requirements and dietary objectives.

Sample Meal Plan (Modify based on preferences and dietary needs)

Day 1:

- Breakfast: Greek yogurt with berries and granola
- lunch: Sandwich with tuna salad on whole-wheat bread with lettuce and tomato
- Snack: Apple slices with almond butter
- Dinner: Baked salmon with roasted vegetables and quinoa

Day 2:

- Breakfast: Eggs scrambled with spinach and whole-wheat bread
- Lunch: Chicken breast salad with mixed greens, avocado, and balsamic vinaigrette
- Snack: Cottage cheese with chopped fruit
- Dinner: Lentil soup with whole-wheat bread

Day 3:

- Breakfast: Oatmeal with cinnamon and nuts
- Lunch: Turkey and vegetable wrap on a whole-wheat tortilla
- Snack: Hummus coupled with carrot sticks and cucumber slices
- Dinner: Shrimp stir-fry with brown rice and broccoli

Day 4:

- Breakfast: Banana, spinach, and protein powder smoothie
- Lunch: Leftover lentil soup with a side salad
- Snack: Yogurt with sliced berries and chia seeds
- Dinner: Baked chicken breast with sweet potato and green beans

Day 5:

- Breakfast: Whole-wheat pancakes with blueberries and maple syrup
- Lunch: Tuna salad lettuce wraps
- Snack: Sliced bell peppers with guacamole
- Dinner: Vegetarian chili with cornbread

Day 6:

- Breakfast: Eggs Benedict with whole-wheat English muffins
- Lunch: Leftover vegetarian chili
- Snack: Popcorn with a sprinkle of parmesan cheese
- Dinner: Grilled salmon with roasted asparagus and brown rice

Day 7:

- Breakfast: French toast with fruit and ricotta cheese

- Lunch: Chicken Caesar salad with whole-grain croutons
- Snack: Trail mix with nuts, seeds, and dried fruit
- Dinner: Grilled steak with grilled vegetables and quinoa

Meal Planning Tips

- Plan your meals ahead of time to ensure you have healthy options on hand and to avoid making poor choices when hungry.
- Cook in large amounts of protein, grains, and veggies to make it easier to prepare meals throughout the week.
- Repurpose leftovers: Repurposing leftovers into new meals saves time and reduces food waste.
- Include spices and herbs: Spices and herbs may bring flavor and diversity to your meals without depending on harmful add-ons.
- Stock up on nutritious snacks: Having fruits, veggies, nuts, and yogurt on hand helps to suppress cravings and encourages healthy eating.

CONCLUSION

Congratulations! You've arrived at the last page of your 28-day fitness plan. But this isn't the conclusion of your narrative; it's the spectacular start of a new you.

Take a minute to ponder the trip you've just begun. Recall that first day, those hesitant steps, the strange soreness in your muscles? Now contrast that with your newfound energy rushing through your body, your sudden confidence in your stride, and your newfound delight in simple actions. You've tested your limitations, accepted challenges, and discovered a strength you didn't know you had.

This book was more than simply an exercise routine; it was a compass pointing you in the direction of a better, happier self. When feelings of doubt whispered in your ear, it was a supporting hand on your back pulling you on. It was a community of peers cheering you on from the side-lines, sharing your successes and failures.

And now that you've arrived at the finish line, you're not the same person that stepped upon the starting line. You're slimmer, stronger, and more energetic. You walk with purpose, your laughter echoes with increased vigor, and your eyes glitter with the assurance of someone who has overcome their worries and triumphed.

The most fundamental shift, however, is not physical; it is psychological. You've uncovered a fountain of inner strength. You've learned to pay attention to your body, appreciate its limitations, and enjoy its accomplishments. You've recognized the value of tiny, steady actions, recognizing that they lead to huge leaps forward.

This is not the conclusion of your fitness journey; rather, it is the start of a new one. The 28 days have given you the tools and confidence to keep going, to make healthy choices, and to embrace an active lifestyle that becomes an extension of who you are.

Thus, take a step away from the page and into the next chapter of your life. Try new things, push yourself with different routines, and maintain that spark of movement. Remember, the best reward isn't a lower dress size or a flatter tummy; it's the sense of success that comes with realizing you can accomplish anything you set your mind to.

Your Thoughts Empower My Journey

Isn't it always bittersweet to reach the final page? It means the experience has come to an end, but it also means you joined me on it. And for that, I am eternally grateful.

Writing these pages was a labor of love, motivated by the desire for the words to connect, inspire, or create a moment of delight. However, the trip does not end here. Your ideas, comments, and candid criticism are the seeds that will nourish my own growth as a writer.

Thus, if you discovered something in this book that struck a chord with you, whether it was a giggle on one page, a cry on another, or perhaps a sense of connection, I encourage you to share it. A small push of motivation, a meaningful critique, or simply a momentary impression - they all serve as a key compass, guiding me to further explore, better, and seek to produce stories that touch people's hearts.

Every reader's voice is a whisper in the wind, but when combined, they create a tremendous symphony that directs my future moves. Remember that even the slightest ripples may cause large waves to form.

Many thanks for joining us on this adventure. And remember that your voice, no matter how quiet, makes all the difference.

With warm regards.

Senior Fitness Planner

Target:

WEEK 1: BALANCE & COORDINATION

workout	Set	Rep	goal

WEEK 2: UPPER BODY STRENGTH

workout	Set	Rep	goal

WEEK 3: LOWER BODY STRENGTH & FLEXIBILITY

workout	Set	Rep	goal

WEEK4: CORE ENGAGEMENT & CARDIO

workout	Set	Rep	goal

Senior Fitness Planner

Target:

WEEK 1: BALANCE & COORDINATION

workout	Set	Rep	goal

WEEK 2: UPPER BODY STRENGTH

workout	Set	Rep	goal

WEEK 3: LOWER BODY STRENGTH & FLEXIBILITY

workout	Set	Rep	goal

WEEK4: CORE ENGAGEMENT & CARDIO

workout	Set	Rep	goal

Senior Fitness Planner

Target:

WEEK 1: BALANCE & COORDINATION

workout	Set	Rep	goal

WEEK 2: UPPER BODY STRENGTH

workout	Set	Rep	goal

WEEK 3: LOWER BODY STRENGTH & FLEXIBILITY

workout	Set	Rep	goal

WEEK4: CORE ENGAGEMENT & CARDIO

workout	Set	Rep	goal

Senior Fitness Planner

Target:

WEEK 1: BALANCE & COORDINATION

workout	Set	Rep	goal

WEEK 2: UPPER BODY STRENGTH

workout	Set	Rep	goal

WEEK 3: LOWER BODY STRENGTH & FLEXIBILITY

workout	Set	Rep	goal

WEEK4: CORE ENGAGEMENT & CARDIO

workout	Set	Rep	goal

www.ingramcontent.com/pod-product-compliance
Lightning Source LLC
Chambersburg PA
CBHW071112260726
48661CB00006B/2583